Simply

Cookbook 2021

The Ultimate Easy and Healthy Keto Cookbook for

Weight Loss in a simple way!

Brian Geller

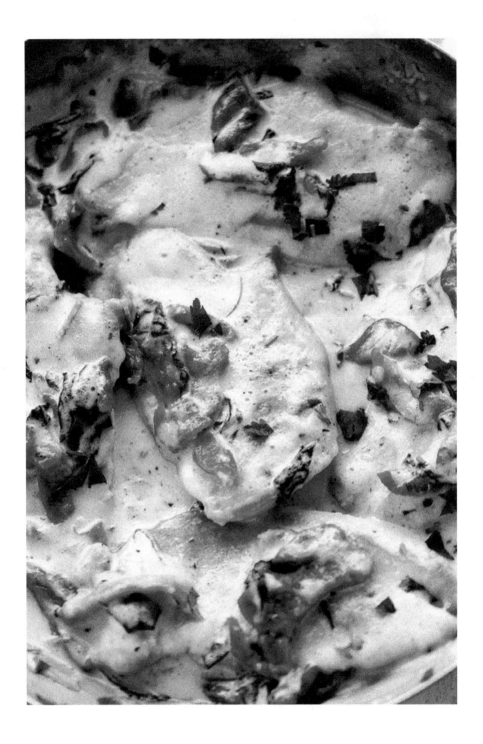

Table of Contents

This declaration is deemed fair and valid by both the American Bar Association and the Committee of Publishers Association and is legally binding throughout the United States.

Furthermore, the transmission, duplication, or reproduction of any of the following work including specific information will be considered an illegal act irrespective of if it is done electronically or in print. This extends to creating a secondary or tertiary copy of the work or a recorded copy and is only allowed with the express written consent from the Publisher. All additional right reserved.

The information in the following pages is broadly considered a truthful and accurate account of facts and as such, any inattention, use, or misuse of the information in question by the reader will render any resulting actions solely under their purview. There are no scenarios in which the publisher or the original author of this work can be in any fashion deemed liable for any hardship or damages that may befall them after undertaking information described herein. Additionally, the information in the following pages is intended only for informational purposes and should thus be thought of as universal. As befitting its nature, it is presented without assurance regarding its prolonged validity or interim quality.

Trademarks that are mentioned are done without written consent and can in no way be considered an endorsement from the trademark holder.

INTRODUCTION

So the Ketogenic Diet is all about reducing the amount of carbohydrates you eat. Does this mean you won't get the kind of energy you need for the day? Of course not! It only means that now, your body has to find other possible sources of energy. Do you know where they will be getting that energy?

Even before we talk about how to do keto – it's important to first consider why this particular diet works. What actually happens to your body to make you lose weight?

As you probably know, the body uses food as an energy source. Everything you eat is turned into energy, so that you can get up and do whatever you need to accomplish for the day. The main energy source is sugar so what happens is that you eat something, the body breaks it down into sugar, and the sugar is processed into energy. Typically, the "sugar" is taken directly from the food you eat so if you eat just the right amount of food, then your body is fueled for the whole day. If you eat too much, then the sugar is stored in your body – hence the accumulation of fat.

But what happens if you eat less food? This is where the Ketogenic Diet comes in. You see, the process of creating sugar from food is usually faster if the food happens to be rich in carbohydrates. Bread, rice, grain, pasta – all of these are carbohydrates and they're the easiest food types to turn into energy.So here's the situation – you are eating less carbohydrates every day. To keep you energetic, the body breaks down the stored fat and turns them into molecules called ketone bodies. The process of turning the fat into ketone bodies is called "Ketosis" and obviously – this is where the name of the Ketogenic Diet comes from. The ketone bodies take the place of glucose in keeping you energetic. As long as you keep your carbohydrates reduced, the body will keep getting its energy from your body fat. The Ketogenic Diet is often praised for its simplicity and when you look at it properly, the process is really straightforward. The Science behind the effectivity of the diet is also well-documented, and has been proven multiple times by different medical fields. For example, an article on Diet Review by Harvard provided a lengthy discussion on how the Ketogenic Diet works and why it is so effective for those who choose to use this diet. But Fat Is the Enemy...Or Is It? No – fat is NOT the enemy. Unfortunately, years of bad science told us that fat is something you have to avoid – but it's actually a very helpful thing for weight loss! Even before we move forward with this book, we'll have to discuss exactly what "healthy fats" are, and why they're actually the good guys. To do this, we need to make a distinction between the different kinds of fat. You've probably heard of them before and it is a little bit confusing at first. We'll try to go through them as simply as possible: Saturated fat. This is the kind you want to avoid. They're also called "solid fat" because each molecule is packed with hydrogen atoms. Simply put, it's the kind of fat that can easily cause a blockage in your body. It can raise cholesterol levels and lead to heart problems or a stroke. Saturated fat is something you can find in meat, dairy products, and other processed food items. Now, you're probably wondering: isn't the Ketogenic Diet packed with saturated fat? The answer is: not necessarily. You'll find later in the recipes given that the Ketogenic Diet promotes primarily unsaturated fat or healthy fat. While there are definitely many meat recipes in the list, most of these recipes contain healthy fat sources.

Unsaturated Fat. These are the ones dubbed as healthy fat. They're the kind of fat you find in avocado, nuts, and other ingredients you usually find in Keto-friendly recipes. They're known to lower blood cholesterol and actually come in two types: polyunsaturated and monounsaturated. Both are good for your body but the benefits slightly vary, depending on what you're consuming.

Bulletproof Tea

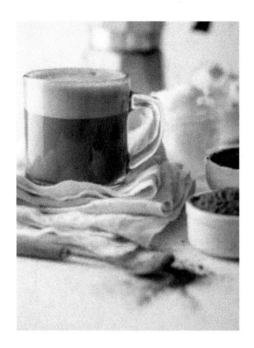

Preparation Time: 5 minutes

Cooking Time: 0 minutes

Servings: 2

Ingredients

- ¼ tsp cinnamon

- 2 cups strong tea

- 2 tbsp. coconut oil

- 2 tbsp. coconut milk

Directions:

1. Distribute tea between two mugs, add remaining ingredients evenly and then stir until blended.

2. Serve.

Nutrition: 151 Calories; 17 g Fats; 0 g Protein; 1 g Net Carb; 0 g Fiber;

Tea with Coconut

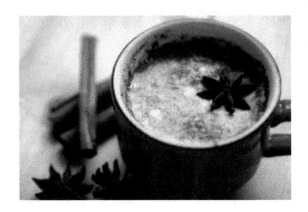

Preparation Time: 10 minutes

Cooking Time: 0 minutes

Servings 2

Ingredients

- 2 tea bags, cinnamon-flavored

- 2 tbsp. MCT oil

- ¼ cup coconut milk, unsweetened

- 2 cups boiling water

Directions:

1. Pour boiling water between two mugs, add a tea into each mug and let them steep for 5 minutes.

2. Meanwhile, take a small saucepan, place it over medium heat, pour in milk and heat for 3 minutes or more until hot.

3. After 5 minutes, remove tea bags from mugs, stir in milk, and MCT oil by using a milk frother until combined and then serve.

Nutrition: 191 Calories; 16 g Fats; 11 g Protein; 2 g Net Carb; 0 g Fiber;

Cauliflower and Egg Plate

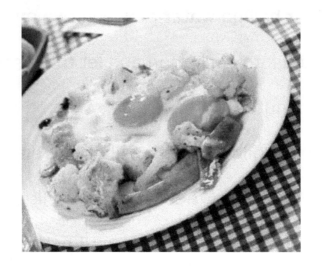

Preparation Time: 5 minutes

Cooking Time: 12 minutes

Servings: 2

Ingredients

- 4 oz. cauliflower florets, chopped

- 1 jalapeno pepper, sliced

- 2 eggs

- 1 ½ tbsp. avocado oil

- Seasoning:

- ¼ tsp salt

- 1/8 tsp ground black pepper

Directions:

1. Take a skillet pan, place it over medium heat, add oil and when hot, add cauliflower florets and jalapeno and then cook for 5 to 7 minutes until tender.

2. Make two spaces in the pan, crack an egg in each space, and then cook for 3 to 4 minutes until eggs have cooked to the desired level.

3. When done, sprinkle salt and black pepper over eggs and then serve.

Nutrition:

191 Calories;

16 g Fats;

11 g Protein;

2 g Net Carb;

0 g Fiber

Butternut Squash and Green Onions with Eggs

Preparation Time: 5 minutes

Cooking Time: 8 minutes

Servings: 2

Ingredients

- 4 oz. butternut squash pieces

- 1 green onion, sliced

- ½ tbsp. butter, unsalted

- 2 tsp grated parmesan cheese

- 2 eggs

- Seasoning:

- ¼ tsp salt

- ¼ tsp ground black pepper

- 1 tsp avocado oil

Directions:

1. Take a skillet pan, place it over medium heat, add butter and oil and when hot, add butternut squash and green onion, season with 1/8 tsp of each salt and black pepper, stir until mixed and cook for 3 to 5 minutes until tender.

2. Make two space in the pan, crack an egg in each space, and sprinkle with cheese, season with remaining salt and black pepper, cover with the lid and cook for 2 to 3 minutes until the egg has cooked to the desired level.

3. Serve.

Nutrition:

191 Calories;

16 g Fats;

11 g Protein;

2 g Net Carb;

0 g Fiber

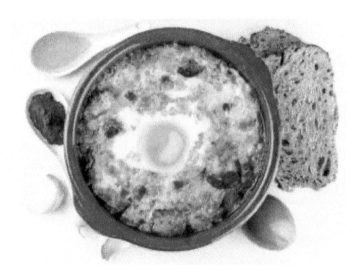

Broccoli, Asparagus and Cheese Frittata

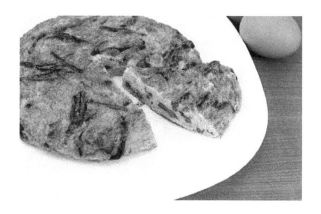

Preparation Time: 5 minutes

Cooking Time: 16 minutes

Servings: 2

Ingredients

- ¼ cup chopped broccoli florets

- 1-ounce asparagus spear cuts

- ½ tsp garlic powder

- 2 tbsp. whipping cream

- 2 eggs

- Seasoning:

- 2 tsp tbsp. avocado oil

- 1/8 tsp salt

- 1/8 tsp ground black pepper

Directions:

1. Turn on the oven, then set it to 350 degrees F and let it preheat.

2. Take a medium bowl, crack eggs in it, add salt, black pepper and cream, whisk until combined and then stir in cheese, set aside until required.

3. Take a medium skillet pan, place it over medium heat, add oil and when hot, add broccoli florets and asparagus, sprinkle with garlic powder, stir until mixed and cook for 3 to 4 minutes until tender.

4. Spread the vegetables evenly in the pan, pour egg mixture over them and cook for 1 to 2 minutes until the mixture begins to firm.

5. Transfer the pan into the oven and then cook for 10 to 12 minutes until frittata has cooked and the top has turned golden brown.

6. When done, cut the frittata into slices and then serve.

Nutrition:

206 Calories;

17 g Fats;

10 g Protein;

2 g Net Carb;

1 g Fiber;

Broccoli and Egg Plate

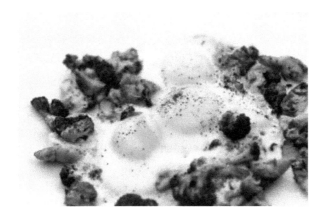

Preparation Time: 5 minutes

Cooking Time: 5 minutes

Servings: 2

Ingredients

- 3 oz. broccoli florets, chopped

- 2 eggs

- 1 tbsp. avocado oil

- ¼ tsp salt

- 1/8 tsp ground black pepper

Directions:

1. Take a heatproof bowl, place broccoli florets in it, cover with a plastic wrap, microwave for 2 minutes, and then drain well.

2. Take a medium skillet pan, place it over medium heat, add oil and when hot, add broccoli florets and cook for 2 minutes until golden brown.

3. Spread broccoli florets evenly in the pan crack eggs in the pan, sprinkle with salt and black pepper, cover with the lid and cook for 2 to 3 minutes until eggs have cooked to the desired level.

4. Serve.

Nutrition: 155 Calories; 12 g Fats; 8 g Protein;

1.6 g Net Carb; 1 g Fiber;

Radish with Fried Eggs

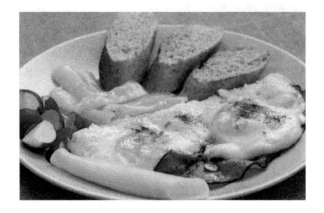

Preparation Time: 5 minutes

Cooking Time: 10 minutes;

Servings: 2

Ingredients

- ½ bunch of radish, diced

- ½ tsp garlic powder

- 1 tbsp. butter

- 1 tbsp. avocado oil

- 2 eggs

- Seasoning:

- 1/3 tsp salt

- ¼ tsp ground black pepper

Directions:

1. Take a medium skillet pan, place it over medium heat, add butter and when it melts, add radish, sprinkle with garlic powder and ¼ tsp salt and cook for 5 minutes until tender.

2. Distribute radish between two plates, then return pan over medium heat, add oil and when hot, crack eggs in it and fry for 2 to 3 minutes until cooked to desired level.

3. Add eggs to the radish and then serve.

Nutrition: 187 Calories; 17 g Fats; 7 g Protein;

0.4 g Net Carb; 0.5 g Fiber;

Sunny Side Up Eggs on Creamed Spinach

Preparation Time: 5 minutes

Cooking Time: 10 minutes

Servings: 2

Ingredients

- 4 oz. of spinach leaves

- 1 tbsp. mustard paste

- 4 tbsp. whipping cream

- 2 eggs

- Seasoning:

- ¼ tsp salt

- ¼ tsp ground black pepper

- ½ tsp dried thyme

- 1 tbsp. avocado oil

Directions:

1. Take a medium skillet pan, place it over high heat, pour in water to cover its bottom, then add spinach, toss until mixed and cook for 2 minutes until spinach wilts.

2. Then drain the spinach by passing it through a sieve placed on a bowl and set it aside.

3. Take a medium saucepan, place it over medium heat, add spinach, mustard, thyme, and cream, stir until mixed and cook for 2 minutes.

4. Then sprinkle black pepper over spinach, stir until mixed and remove the pan from heat.

5. Take a medium skillet pan, place it over medium-high heat, add oil and when hot, crack eggs in it and fry for 3 to 4 minutes until eggs have cooked to the desired level.

6. Divide spinach mixture evenly between two plates, top with a fried egg and then serve.

Nutrition: 280 Calories; 23.3 g Fats; 10.2 g Protein; 2.7 g Net Carb; 2.8 g Fiber;

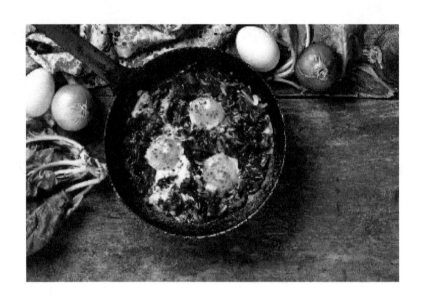

Creamy Kale Baked Eggs

Preparation Time: 10 minutes

Cooking Time: 20 minutes

Servings: 2

Ingredients

- 1 bunch of kale, chopped

- 1-ounce grape tomatoes, halved

- 3 tbsp. whipping cream

- 2 tbsp. sour cream

- 2 eggs

- Seasoning:

- ½ tsp salt

- ½ tsp ground black pepper

- ½ tsp Italian seasoning

- 1 ½ tbsp. butter, unsalted

Directions:

1. Turn on the oven, then set it to 400 degrees F and let it preheat.

2. Meanwhile, take a medium skillet pan, place butter in it, add butter and when it melts, add kale and cook for 2 minutes until wilted

3. Add Italian seasoning, 1/3 tsp each of salt and black pepper, cream and sour cream, then stir until mixed and cook for2 minutes until cheese has melted and the kale has thickened slightly.

4. Take two ramekins, divide creamed kale evenly between them, then top with cherry tomatoes and carefully crack an egg into each ramekin.

5. Sprinkle remaining salt and black pepper on eggs and then bake for 15 minutes until eggs have cooked completely.

6. Serve.

Nutrition:

301.5 Calories;

25.5 g Fats;

9.8 g Protein;

4.3 g Net Carb;

4 g Fiber;

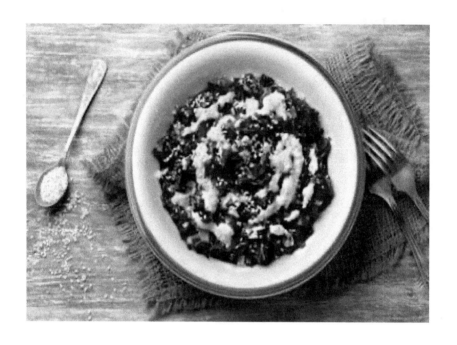

Butter Asparagus with Creamy Eggs

Preparation Time: 5 minutes

Cooking Time: 8 minutes

Servings: 2

Ingredients

- 4 oz. asparagus

- 2 eggs, blended

    1. oz. grated parmesan cheese

- 1-ounce sour cream

- 2 tbsp. butter, unsalted

- Seasoning:

- 1/3 tsp salt

- 1/8 tsp ground black pepper

- ¼ tsp cayenne pepper

- ½ tbsp. avocado oil

Directions:

1. Take a medium skillet pan, place it over medium heat, add butter and when it melts, add blended eggs and then cook for 2 to 3 minutes until scrambled to the desired level; don't overcook.

2. Spoon the scrambled eggs into a food processor, add 1/8 tsp salt, cayenne pepper, sour cream and cheese and then pulse for 1 minute until smooth.

3. Return skillet pan over medium heat, add oil and when hot, add asparagus, season with black pepper and remaining salt, toss until mixed and

cook for 3 minutes or more until roasted.

4. Distribute asparagus between two plates, add egg mixture, and then serve.

Nutrition:

338 Calories;

28.5 g Fats;

14.4 g Protein;

4.7 g Net Carb;

1.2 g Fiber;

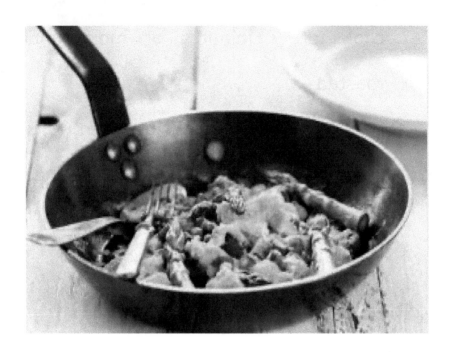

Spinach Egg Muffins

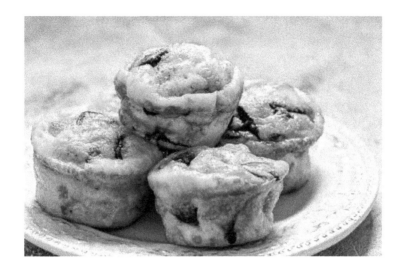

Preparation Time: 5 minutes

Cooking Time: 10 minutes

Servings: 2

Ingredients

- ½ cups chopped spinach

- 1/8 tsp dried basil

- 1/8 tsp garlic powder

- 2 large eggs

- 3 tbsp. grated Parmesan cheese

- Seasoning:

- ¼ tsp of sea salt

- 1/8 tsp ground black pepper

Directions:

1. Turn on the oven, then set it to 400 degrees F, and let preheat.

2. Meanwhile, place eggs in a bowl, season with salt and black pepper and whisk until blended.

3. Add garlic and basil, whisk in mixed and then stir in spinach and cheese until combined.

4. Take two silicone muffin cups, grease them with reserved bacon greased, fill

them evenly with prepared egg mixture and bake for 8 to 10 minutes until the top has nicely browned.

5. Serve.

Nutrition: 55 Calories; 3.5 g Fats; 4.5 g Protein; 0.4 g Net Carb; 0.2 g Fiber;

Broccoli and Egg Muffin

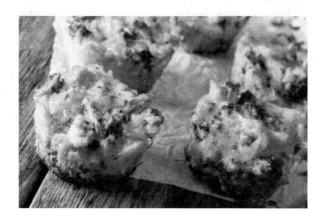

Preparation Time: 10 minutes;

Cooking Time: 10 minutes

Servings: 2

Ingredients

- ¼ cup broccoli florets, steamed, chopped

- 2 tbsp. grated cheddar cheese

- 1/16 tsp dried thyme

- 1/16 tsp garlic powder

- 1 egg

- Seasoning:

- ¼ tsp salt

- 1/8 tsp ground black pepper

Directions:

1. Turn on the oven, then set it to 400 degrees F and let it preheat.

2. Meanwhile, take two silicone muffin cups, grease them with oil, and evenly fill them with broccoli and cheese.

3. Crack the egg in a bowl, add garlic powder, thyme, salt, and black pepper, whisk well, then evenly pour the mixture into muffin cups and bake for 8 to 10 minutes until done.

4. Serve.

Nutrition: 76 Calories; 5.1 g Fats; 5.7 g Protein; 1.2 g Net Carb; 0.7 g Fiber;

Jalapeno and Cheese Egg Muffins

Preparation Time: 10 minutes

Cooking Time: 15 minutes

Servings: 2

Ingredients

- 1 jalapeno pepper, diced

- 2 tbsp. sliced green onions

- 2 tbsp. grated parmesan cheese

- 1 tsp all-purpose seasoning

- 2 eggs

- Seasoning:

- 1/3 tsp salt

- ¼ tsp ground black pepper

Directions:

1. Turn on the oven, then set it to 375 degrees F, and let it preheat.

2. Meanwhile, take two silicone muffin cups, grease with oil, and evenly fill them with cheese, jalapeno pepper, and green onion.

3. Crack eggs in a bowl, season with salt, black pepper, and all-purpose seasoning, whisk well, then evenly pour the mixture into muffin cups and bake for 15 to 20 minutes or until the top is slightly brown and muffins have puffed up.

4. Serve.

Nutrition: 108 Calories; 7.1 g Fats; 8.9 g Protein; 1.8 g Net Carb; 0.4 g Fiber;

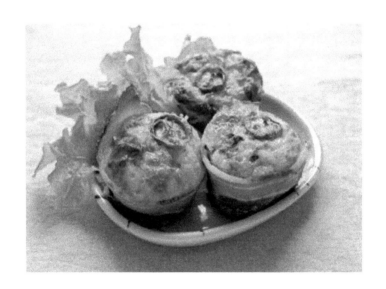

Cheesy Tomato and Olive Muffins

Preparation Time: 10 minutes

Cooking Time: 12 minutes

Servings: 2

Ingredients

- 4 1/3 tbsp. almond flour

- ½ tbsp. coconut flour

- 1/3 tbsp. chopped tomato

- 1/3 tbsp. sliced green olives

- 2 tbsp. sour cream

- Seasoning:

- 1/8 tsp baking powder

- 2/3 tbsp. avocado oil

- 3 tbsp. grated parmesan cheese

- ½ of egg

Directions:

1. Turn on the oven, then set it to 320 degrees F and let it preheat.

2. Meanwhile, take a medium bowl, place flours in it, and stir in the baking powder until mixed.

3. Add eggs along with sour cream and oil, whisk until blended and then fold in cheese, tomato, and olives until just mixed.

4. Take two silicone muffin cups, add the prepared batter in it evenly and then bake for 10 to 12 minutes until cooked but slightly moist in the middle.

5. When done, let muffin cools for 5 minutes, then take them out and serve.

Nutrition:

256 Calories;

23.5 g Fats;

8.7 g Protein;

1 g Net Carb;

1.8 g Fiber;

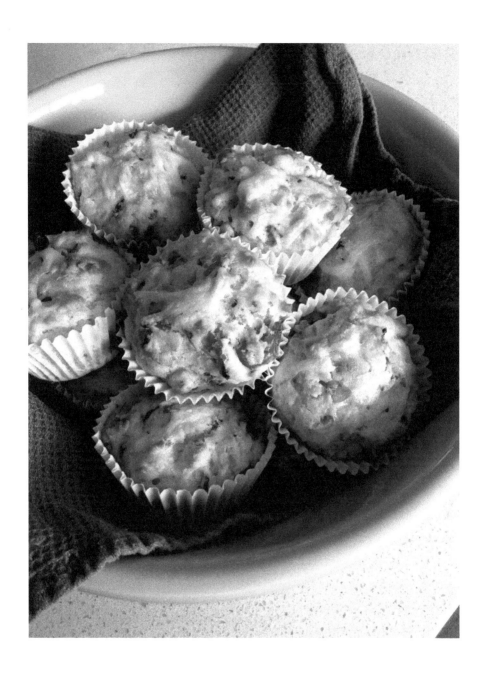

Buttery Broccoli and Bacon

Preparation Time: 5 minutes

Cooking Time: 12 minutes

Servings: 2

Ingredients

1 slice of turkey bacon

1 cup chopped broccoli florets

1/8 tsp garlic powder

¼ tsp Italian seasoning

¼ tbsp. unsalted butter

Seasoning:

1/8 tsp salt

1/8 tsp ground black pepper

Directions:

1. Take a medium skillet pan, place it over high heat, add bacon slice and cook for 3 to 5 minutes until crispy.

2. Transfer bacon to a cutting board and then chop it into small pieces.

3. Reduce the heat to medium-low level, add broccoli florets into the pan, stir well into the bacon grease, add butter, then toss until mixed and cook for 5 minutes until tender.

4. Season the broccoli florets with salt, black pepper, and Italian seasoning, add chopped bacon, stir well and cook for 2 minutes until thoroughly heated.

5. Serve.

Nutrition:

77 Calories;

5 g Fats;

5 g Protein;

1 g Net Carb;

2 g Fiber;

Broccoli Salad with Bacon

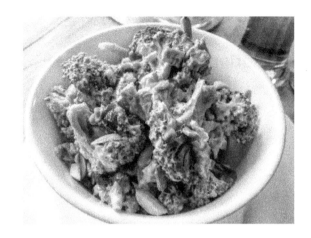

Preparation Time: 5 minutes

Cooking Time: 0 minutes

Servings: 2

Ingredients

- 1 cup broccoli florets, chopped

- 4 tbsp. whipped topping

- 2 tbsp. shredded cheddar cheese

- 3 slices of turkey bacon, cooked, chopped

- 1/3 tsp garlic powder

- Seasoning:

- 1/8 tsp salt

- 1/8 tsp dried parsley

Directions:

1. Take a medium bowl, place whipped topping in it, whisk in garlic powder and parsley, and then fold in broccoli florets.

2. Top with bacon and cheddar cheese and serve.

Nutrition: 119 Calories; 10 g Fats; 3.5 g Protein; 2 g Net Carb; 0.5 g Fiber;

BEEF

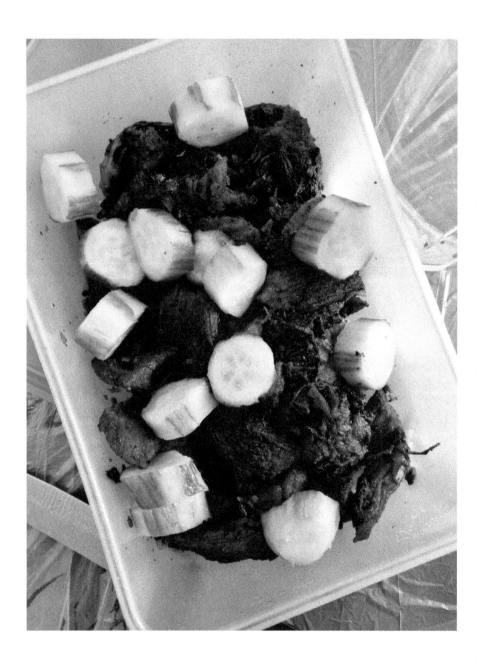

Beef and Broccoli

Preparation Time: 5 minutes

Cooking Time: 10 minutes

Servings: 2

Ingredients

- 6 slices of beef roast, cut into strips

- 1 scallion, chopped

- 3 oz. broccoli florets, chopped

- 1 tbsp. avocado oil

- 1 tbsp. butter, unsalted

- Seasoning:

- ¼ tsp salt

- 1/8 tsp ground black pepper

- 1 ½ tbsp. soy sauce

- 3 tbsp. chicken broth

Directions:

1. Take a medium skillet pan, place it over medium heat, add oil and when hot, add beef strips and cook for 2 minutes until hot.

2. Transfer beef to a plate, add scallion to the pan, then add butter and cook for 3 minutes until tender.

3. Add remaining ingredients, stir until mixed, switch heat to the low level and simmer for 3 to 4 minutes until broccoli is tender.

4. Return beef to the pan, stir until well combined and cook for 1 minute.

5. Serve.

Nutrition:

245 Calories;

15.7 g Fats;

21.6 g Protein;

1.7 g Net Carb;

1.3 g Fiber;

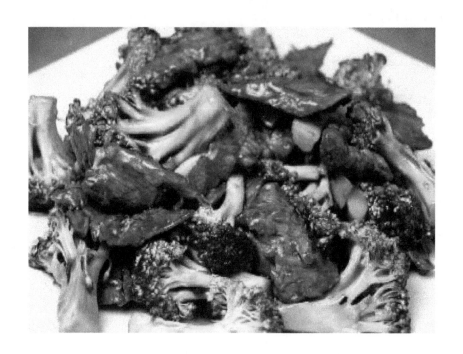

Beef with Cabbage Noodles

Preparation Time: 5 minutes

Cooking Time: 18 minutes

Servings: 2

Ingredients

- 4 oz. ground beef

- 1 cup chopped cabbage

- 4 oz. tomato sauce

- ½ tsp minced garlic

- ½ cup of water

- Seasoning:

- ½ tbsp. coconut oil

- ½ tsp salt

- ¼ tsp Italian seasoning

- 1/8 tsp dried basil

Directions:

1. Take a skillet pan, place it over medium heat, add oil and when hot, add beef and cook for 5 minutes until nicely browned.

2. Meanwhile, prepare the cabbage and for it, slice the cabbage into thin shred.

3. When the beef has cooked, add garlic, season with salt, basil, and Italian seasoning, stir well and continue cooking for 3 minutes until beef has thoroughly cooked.

4. Pour in tomato sauce and water, stir well and bring the mixture to boil.

5. Then reduce heat to medium-low level, add cabbage, stir well until well mixed and

simmer for 3 to 5 minutes until cabbage is softened, covering the pan.

6. Uncover the pan and continue simmering the beef until most of the cooking liquid has evaporated.

7. Serve.

Nutrition:

188.5 Calories;

12.5 g Fats;

15.5 g Protein;

2.5 g Net Carb;

1 g Fiber;

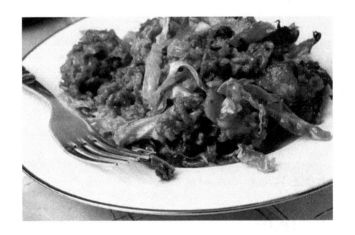

Garlic Herb Beef Roast

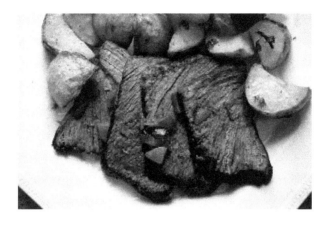

Preparation Time: 5 minutes

Cooking Time: 10 minutes

Servings: 2

Ingredients

- 6 slices of beef roast

- ½ tsp garlic powder

- 1/3 tsp dried thyme

- ¼ tsp dried rosemary

- 2 tbsp. butter, unsalted

- Seasoning:

- 1/3 tsp salt

- 1/4 tsp ground black pepper

Directions:

1. Prepare the spice mix and for this, take a small bowl, place garlic powder, thyme, rosemary, salt, and black pepper and then stir until mixed.

2. Sprinkle spice mix on the beef roast.

3. Take a medium skillet pan, place it over medium heat, add butter and when it melts, add beef roast and then cook for 5 to 8 minutes until golden brown and cooked.

4. Serve.

Nutrition: 140 Calories; 12.7 g Fats; 5.5 g

Protein; 0.1 g Net Carb; 0.2 g Fiber;

Garlicky Steaks with Rosemary

Preparation Time: 25 minutes

Cooking Time: 12 minutes

Servings: 2

Ingredients

- 2 beef steaks
- 1/4 of a lime, juiced
- 1 ½ tsp garlic powder
- ¾ tsp dried rosemary
- 2 ½ tbsp. avocado oil
- Seasoning:
- ½ tsp salt
- ¼ tsp ground black pepper

Directions:

1. Prepare steaks, and for this, sprinkle garlic powder on all sides of steak.

2. Take a shallow dish, place 1 ½ tbsp. oil and lime juice in it, whisk until combined, add steaks, turn to coat and let it marinate for 20 minutes at room temperature.

3. Then take a griddle pan, place it over medium-high heat and grease it with remaining oil.

4. Season marinated steaks with salt and black pepper, add to the griddle pan and cook for 7 to 12 minutes until cooked to the desired level.

5. When done, wrap steaks in foil for 5 minutes, then cut into slices across the grain.

6. Sprinkle rosemary over steaks slices and then serve.

Nutrition:

213 Calories;

13 g Fats;

22 g Protein;

1 g Net Carb;

0 g Fiber;

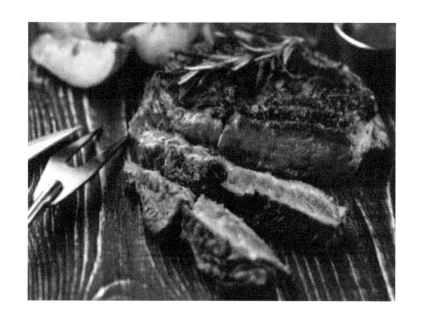

Roast Beef and Mozzarella Plate

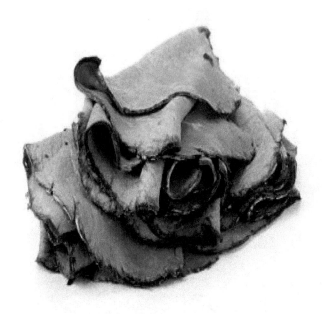

Preparation Time: 5 minutes

Cooking Time: 0 minutes

Servings: 2

Ingredients

- 4 slices of roast beef

- ½ ounce chopped lettuce

- 1 avocado, pitted

- 2 oz. mozzarella cheese, cubed

- ½ cup mayonnaise

- Seasoning:

- ¼ tsp salt

- 1/8 tsp ground black pepper

- 2 tbsp. avocado oil

Directions:

1. Scoop out flesh from avocado and divide it evenly between two plates.

2. Add slices of roast beef, lettuce, and cheese and then sprinkle with salt and black pepper.

3. Serve with avocado oil and mayonnaise.

Nutrition: 267.7 Calories; 24.5 g Fats; 9.5 g Protein; 1.5 g Net Carb; 2 g Fiber;

Sprouts Stir-fry with Kale, Broccoli, and Beef

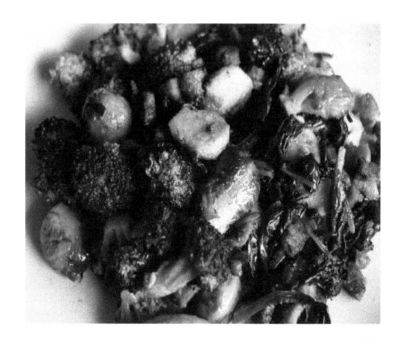

Preparation Time: 5 minutes

Cooking Time: 8 minutes

Servings: 2

Ingredients

- 3 slices of beef roast, chopped

- 2 oz. Brussels sprouts, halved

- 4 oz. broccoli florets

- 3 oz. kale

- 1 ½ tbsp. butter, unsalted

- 1/8 tsp red pepper flakes

- Seasoning:

- ¼ tsp garlic powder

- ¼ tsp salt

- 1/8 tsp ground black pepper

Directions:

1. Take a medium skillet pan, place it over medium heat, add ¾ tbsp. butter and when it melts, add broccoli florets and sprouts, sprinkle with garlic powder, and cook for 2 minutes.

2. Season vegetables with salt and red pepper flakes, add chopped beef, stir until mixed and continue cooking for 3 minutes until browned on one side.

3. Then add kale along with remaining butter, flip the vegetables and cook for 2 minutes until kale leaves wilts.

4. Serve.

Nutrition: 125 Calories; 9.4 g Fats; 4.8 g Protein; 1.7 g Net Carb; 2.6 g Fiber;

Beef and Vegetable Skillet

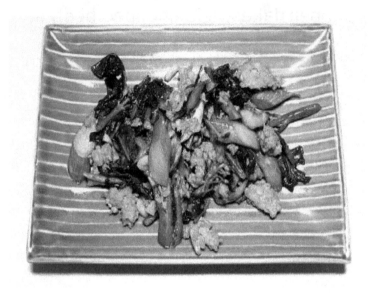

Preparation Time: 5 minutes

Cooking Time: 15 minutes

Servings: 2

Ingredients

- 3 oz. spinach, chopped

- ½ pound ground beef

- 2 slices of bacon, diced

- 2 oz. chopped asparagus

- Seasoning:

- 3 tbsp. coconut oil

- 2 tsp dried thyme

- 2/3 tsp salt

- ½ tsp ground black pepper

Directions:

1. Take a skillet pan, place it over medium heat, add oil and when hot, add beef and bacon and cook for 5 to 7 minutes until slightly browned.

2. Then add asparagus and spinach, sprinkle with thyme, stir well and cook for 7 to 10 minutes until thoroughly cooked.

3. Season skillet with salt and black pepper and serve.

Nutrition: 332.5 Calories; 26 g Fats; 23.5 g Protein; 1.5 g Net Carb; 1 g Fiber;

Beef, Pepper and Green Beans Stir-fry

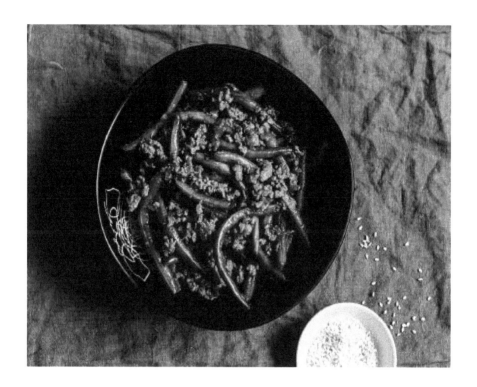

Preparation Time: 5 minutes

Cooking Time: 18 minutes

Servings: 2

Ingredients

- 6 oz. ground beef

- 2 oz. chopped green bell pepper

- 4 oz. green beans

- 3 tbsp. grated cheddar cheese

- Seasoning:

- ½ tsp salt

- ¼ tsp ground black pepper

- ¼ tsp paprika

Directions:

1. Take a skillet pan, place it over medium heat, add ground beef and cook for 4 minutes until slightly browned.

2. Then add bell pepper and green beans, season with salt, paprika, and black pepper, stir well and continue cooking for 7 to 10 minutes until beef and vegetables have cooked through.

3. Sprinkle cheddar cheese on top, then transfer pan under the broiler and cook for 2 minutes until cheese has melted and the top is golden brown.

4. Serve.

Nutrition: 282.5 Calories; 17.6 g Fats; 26.1 g Protein; 2.9 g Net Carb; 2.1 g Fiber;

Roast Beef and Vegetable Plate

Preparation Time: 10 minutes

Cooking Time: 10 minutes

Servings: 2

Ingredients

- 2 scallions, chopped in large pieces

- 1 ½ tbsp. coconut oil

- 4 thin slices of roast beef

- 4 oz. cauliflower and broccoli mix

- 1 tbsp. butter, unsalted

- Seasoning:

- 1/2 tsp salt

- 1/3 tsp ground black pepper

- 1 tsp dried parsley

Directions:

1. Turn on the oven, then set it to 400 degrees F, and let it preheat.
2. Take a baking sheet, grease it with oil, place slices of roast beef on one side, and top with butter.
3. Take a separate bowl, add cauliflower and broccoli mix, add scallions, drizzle with oil, season with remaining salt and black pepper, toss until coated and then spread vegetables on the empty side of the baking sheet.

4. Bake for 5 to 7 minutes until beef is nicely browned and vegetables are tender-crisp, tossing halfway.

5. Distribute beef and vegetables between two plates and then serve.

Nutrition:

313 Calories;

26 g Fats;

15.6 g Protein;

2.8 g Net Carb;

1.9 g Fiber;

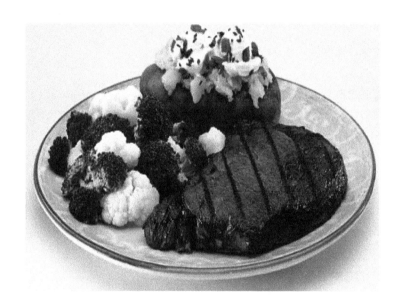

Dijon Celery Salad

Preparation Time: 10 minutes

Cooking Time: 0 minutes

Servings: 4

Ingredients:

- 5 teaspoons stevia

- ½ cup lemon juice

- 1/3 cup Dijon mustard

- 2/3 cup olive oil

- Black pepper to the taste

- 2 apples, cored, peeled and cubed

- 1 bunch celery and leaves, roughly chopped

- ¾ cup walnuts, chopped

Directions:

1. In a salad bowl, mix celery and its leaves with apple pieces and walnuts.

2. Add black pepper, lemon juice, mustard, stevia and olive oil, whisk well, add to your salad, toss, divide into small cups and serve as a snack.

Nutrition:

Calories 125

Fat 2

Fiber 2

Carbs 7

Protein 7

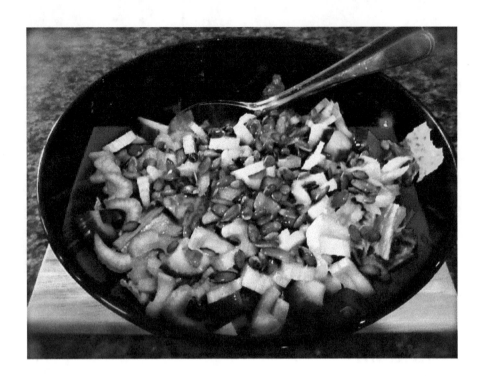

Napa Cabbage Slaw

Preparation Time: 10 minutes

Cooking Time: 0 minutes

Servings: 4

Ingredients:

- ½ cup of red bell pepper, cut into thin strips
- 1 carrot, grated
- 4 cups Napa cabbage, shredded
- 3 green onions, chopped
- 1 tablespoon olive oil
- 2 teaspoons ginger, grated
- ½ teaspoon red pepper flakes, crushed
- 3 tablespoons balsamic vinegar
- 1 tablespoon coconut aminos
- 3 tablespoons low-fat peanut butter

Directions:

1. In a salad bowl, mix bell pepper with carrot, cabbage and onions and toss.

2. Add oil, ginger, pepper flakes, vinegar, aminos and peanut butter, toss, divide into small cups and serve.

Nutrition:

Calories 160

Fat 10

Fiber 3

Carbs 10

Protein 5

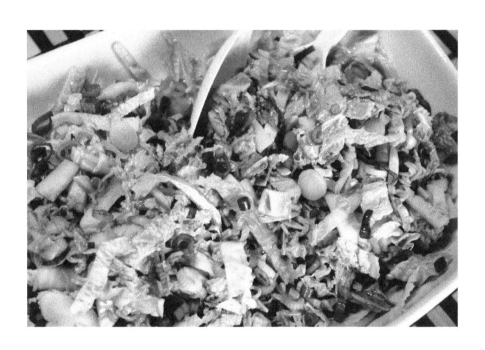

CONCLUSION

The things to watch out for when coming off keto are weight gain, bloating, more energy, and feeling hungry. The weight gain is nothing to freak out over; perhaps, you might not even gain any. It all depends on your diet, how your body processes carbs, and, of course, water weight. The length of your keto diet is a significant factor in how much weight you have lost, which is caused by the reduction of carbs. The bloating will occur because of the reintroduction of fibrous foods and your body getting used to digesting them again. The bloating van lasts for a few days to a few weeks. You will feel like you have more energy because carbs break down into glucose, which is the body's primary source of fuel. You may also notice better brain function and the ability to work out more.

Whether you have met your weight loss goals, your life changes, or you simply want to eat whatever you want again. You cannot just suddenly start consuming carbs again for it will shock your system. Have an idea of what you want to allow back into your consumption slowly. Be familiar with portion sizes and stick to that amount of carbs for the first few times you eat post-keto. Start with non-processed carbs like whole grain, beans, and fruits. Start slow and see how your body responds before resolving to add carbs one meal at a time.

The ketogenic diet is the ultimate tool you can use to plan your future. Can you picture being more involved, more productive and efficient, and more relaxed and energetic? That future is possible for you, and it does not have to be a complicated process to achieve that vision. You can choose right now to be healthier and slimmer and more fulfilled tomorrow. It is possible with the ketogenic diet. It does not just improve your physical health but your mental and emotional health as well. This diet improves your health holistically. Do not give up now as there will be quite a few days where you may think to yourself, "Why am I doing this?" and to answer that, simply focus on the goals you wish to achieve. A good diet enriched with all the proper nutrients is our best shot of achieving an active metabolism and efficient lifestyle. A lot of people think that the Keto diet is simply for people who are interested in losing weight. You will find that it is quite the opposite. There are intense keto diets where only 5 percent of the diet comes from carbs, 20 percent is from protein, and 75 percent is from fat. But even a modified version of this which involves consciously choosing foods low in carbohydrate and high in healthy fats is good enough. Thanks for reading this book. I hope it has provided you with enough insight to get you going. Don't put off getting started. The sooner you begin this diet, the sooner you'll start to notice an improvement in your health and well-being.

CPSIA information can be obtained
at www.ICGtesting.com
Printed in the USA
LVHW081135080721
692066LV00003B/82